Naoko Morisaki

The oral conditions and Health-related QOL among dependent elderly

AF168229

Naoko Morisaki

The oral conditions and Health-related QOL among dependent elderly

LAP LAMBERT Academic Publishing

Impressum / Imprint
Bibliografische Information der Deutschen Nationalbibliothek: Die Deutsche
Nationalbibliothek verzeichnet diese Publikation in der Deutschen
Nationalbibliografie; detaillierte bibliografische Daten sind im Internet über
http://dnb.d-nb.de abrufbar.
Alle in diesem Buch genannten Marken und Produktnamen unterliegen
warenzeichen-, marken- oder patentrechtlichem Schutz bzw. sind
Warenzeichen oder eingetragene Warenzeichen der jeweiligen Inhaber. Die
Wiedergabe von Marken, Produktnamen, Gebrauchsnamen, Handelsnamen,
Warenbezeichnungen u.s.w. in diesem Werk berechtigt auch ohne besondere
Kennzeichnung nicht zu der Annahme, dass solche Namen im Sinne der
Warenzeichen- und Markenschutzgesetzgebung als frei zu betrachten wären
und daher von jedermann benutzt werden dürften.

Bibliographic information published by the Deutsche Nationalbibliothek: The
Deutsche Nationalbibliothek lists this publication in the Deutsche
Nationalbibliografie; detailed bibliographic data are available in the Internet
at http://dnb.d-nb.de.
Any brand names and product names mentioned in this book are subject to
trademark, brand or patent protection and are trademarks or registered
trademarks of their respective holders. The use of brand names, product
names, common names, trade names, product descriptions etc. even without
a particular marking in this work is in no way to be construed to mean that
such names may be regarded as unrestricted in respect of trademark and
brand protection legislation and could thus be used by anyone.

Coverbild / Cover image: www.ingimage.com

Verlag / Publisher:
LAP LAMBERT Academic Publishing
ist ein Imprint der / is a trademark of
OmniScriptum GmbH & Co. KG
Heinrich-Böcking-Str. 6-8, 66121 Saarbrücken, Deutschland / Germany
Email: info@lap-publishing.com

Herstellung: siehe letzte Seite /
Printed at: see last page
ISBN: 978-3-659-34108-3

Contents

I. Introduction

Given the prolonged mean life expectancy and decrease in birth rates, population aging is progressing worldwide. In developed countries, in 1998, the number of elderly people had already exceeded the number of children, a phenomenon that is estimated to occur worldwide in the year 2045. The global population aged 60 years or older increased by 3.5-fold from 205 million to 737 million between the years 1950 and 2009, after which it continued to increase at an annual rate of 1.2%, and is predicted to further increase by 3-fold to 2 billion in 2050. Particularly in developed countries, the proportion of people aged 60 years or older is expected to increase from 20% in 2009 to approximately 30% in 2050. Currently, Japan is ranked first worldwide in terms of the population aging rate.

The number of elderly people in Japan has increased considerably and has been accompanied by an increase in the number of elderly people requiring nursing care. In Japan, elderly people requiring nursing care tend to spend their daily lives in their homes rather than in nursing care facilities, a traditional practice, and as a result, additional measures need to be taken in regard to elderly who community-dwelling dependent elderly persons. Compared to institutionalized elderly people, elderly people who live at home have less severe illnesses and can live their daily lives somewhat independently, even if they suffer from some type of disorder. The percentage of people requiring mild long-term care has become relatively high. In Japan, more than 80% of people requiring mild long-term care use home care services provided through the long-term care insurance system; as a result, home care services for elderly people living at home need improvement.

For the elderly, the oral cavity is an organ that directly supports nutrition, and the act of eating and swallowing food through the oral cavity comprises a series of processes that consist of incorporating food servings as nutrients needed to remain alive and delivering them properly to the stomach. This is among the essential daily bodily functions that are indispensable for maintaining life. Whereas most bodily functions decline with age, previous studies[1][2] have shown that in the elderly, deteriorations of the oral environment and oral functions are factors that contribute to the occurrence of severe conditions such as pneumonia and malnutrition and factors that are deeply involved in the physical and vital prognosis.

From a global perspective, pneumonia is a major cause of death in children, and can be severe and life threatening in people with low immunity or reserve capacities. In Japan, although pneumonia is the third-ranked cause of death in people of all

3

ages, the number of deaths due to pneumonia has increased annually particularly among the elderly. In the year 2010, elderly people aged 65 years and older accounted for 96.6% of deaths due to pneumonia. Among elderly people requiring nursing care, pneumonia was the most common cause of death, accounting for 30% of all cases. In fact, among deaths occurring in elderly care facilities, the highest number were due to pneumonia[3]. In elderly subjects, most cases of pneumonia are classified as dysphagia pneumonia, which is caused by pulmonary dysphagia; the percentage of dysphagia pneumonia cases increases with age. A national survey conducted in Japan showed that 80% of pneumonia cases occurring in people aged 70 years or older were dysphagia pneumonia[4]. Bacteria in the oral cavity, which are the causal microorganisms of dysphagia pneumonia, flow into the respiratory tract along with saliva and food when pulmonary dysphagia occurs, leading to pneumonia. However, evidence has shown that elderly people requiring nursing care harbor larger numbers of bacteria in their oral cavities and have poorly maintained oral environments. In addition, deterioration of the oral cavity condition contributes to malnutrition and even in Japan, a developed country, 20–40% of elderly people requiring nursing care are considered at risk of malnutrition[5]. Previous reports based on surveys of elderly subjects requiring nursing care have shown that regarding malnutrition, the nutritional status was associated with serum albumin levels, weight loss, tongue pressure[6], or with subcutaneous fat thickness associated with the triceps muscle and the swallowing function[2]; in other words, malnutrition in elderly subjects requiring nursing care is associated with oral functioning.

Despite progress in elucidating the association between the vital prognosis, including physical health, and the oral cavity condition, other reports have shown an association between oral health and psychological conditions. According to reports based on studies of institutionalized elderly subjects, oral functioning not only affected physical health, but was also associated with psychological functions such as the oral cavity-related quality of life (QOL)[7] and volition[8]. In addition, reports on elderly subjects who lived their daily lives independently in regional communities also suggested that the dysphagia risk resulting from deteriorated oral function associated significantly with "mental health" on a sub-scale of the SF-8, an evaluation index for health-related QOL[9]. In elderly subjects, especially those at advanced ages, it is important to determine how to maintain or improve the daily QOL and in consideration of elderly care in the future, the oral cavity condition might also be very meaningful in terms of its association with the QOL, in addition to its involvement with dietary life and physical health.

4

In a study of oral functioning in independent elderly subjects, Miura et al.[9] reported that 30% of the subjects were at risk of a decreased swallowing function and that elderly subjects living at home were thought to exhibit deterioration of the oral cavity condition. In addition, among elderly subjects who live at home while suffering from some type of disorder and thus require long-term nursing care, a considerable number have been estimated to be at risk of experiencing oral function deterioration and related needs. However, additional epidemiological studies on the oral cavity condition of elderly subjects requiring nursing care have been conducted among institutionalized elderly subjects, and comparatively, case reports of dependent community-dwelling elderly persons remain insufficient; therefore, the findings need to be accumulated. To improve oral care among elderly people receiving long-term care at home, an understanding of the needs pertaining to oral care is essential and indispensable, and in order to determine and analyze needs, the studies should not be limited to aspects related to the intra-oral environment alone, but might also include oral functions.

Therefore, to examine the oral care-related needs among community-dwelling dependent elderly persons elderly in Japan, this study aimed to elucidate the oral cavity condition from the perspectives of oral functioning and the intra-oral environment and to analyze the association between the oral cavity condition and health-related QOL.

II. Methods

1. Research methodology

A questionnaire survey and field survey on the oral cavity conditions were conducted from 2013 to 2014.

2. Study participants

This study included elderly subjects aged 65 years or older who lived at home in Hyogo prefecture (Japan) and required nursing care. The majority of elderly subjects receiving long-term home care in Japan use daycare services during the daytime. Accordingly, the surveys included dependent community-dwelling elderly persons and attending daycare service facilities. From among the 440 elderly subjects attending 7 daycare service facilities that agreed to collaborate with us in this study, the participants comprised 225 individuals with stable physical and psychological conditions who were able to participate in daily conversations to the extent necessary for the survey and who consented to participate in this study.

3. Survey items and evaluation methods

1) Basic status

The following were surveyed: age, sex, cognitive function, activities of daily living (ADL), nutritional status, and current disease.

Data pertaining to age, sex, level of care needed, and cognitive function were obtained from the daycare service facilities attended by the participants. The methods used by the facilities to evaluate cognitive function comprised the mini-mental state examination (MMSE)[10], Hasegawa's dementia scale (HDS-R)[11], and the mental status questionnaire (MSQ)[12]; based on those evaluations, individuals who were determined to have a severe cognitive function impairment were excluded from participation.

Regarding ADL, a questionnaire survey using the ADL20 evaluation method[13], a comprehensive ADL evaluation index, was conducted. On this scale, the degree of independence was calculated based the participants' responses to the 20 items pertaining to activities of daily living and was classified as 1 of 4 levels: "full assistance: 0 points", "monitoring or partial assistance: 1 point", "independence with use of an assisting device: 2 points", "full independence: 3 points". A higher total point value indicated a higher degree of independence.

Regarding the nutritional status, the mini-nutritional assessment short-form

(MNA-SF)[14)15)], which was designed for elderly subjects aged 65 years or older, was used. This method used the following as evaluation items: dietary intake conditions, weight loss, walking conditions, acute physical and psychological stress, cognitive function, depression, and body mass index (BMI). The malnutrition index was calculated as the sum of points from each item; a total point value between 12 and 14 was considered good nutritional status, between 8 and 11 was considered at risk of malnutrition, and between 0 and 7 was considered malnutrition. Data pertaining to stature and body weight, which were necessary for BMI calculations, were obtained from the facilities.

2) Health-related QOL

   SF-8 [16)] was used for the evaluation of health-related QOL, as it facilitated measurements of QOL in terms of 8 health-related areas. The 8 areas were as follows: physical functioning (PF), role physical (RP), bodily pain (BP), general health (GH), vitality (VT), social functioning (SF), role emotional (RE), and mental health (MH). The SF-8 evaluation was based on the SF-8 Japanese version (Figure 1) and standard edition evaluation sheet. Each scale score was calculated based the national standard value, using the SF-8 scoring program.

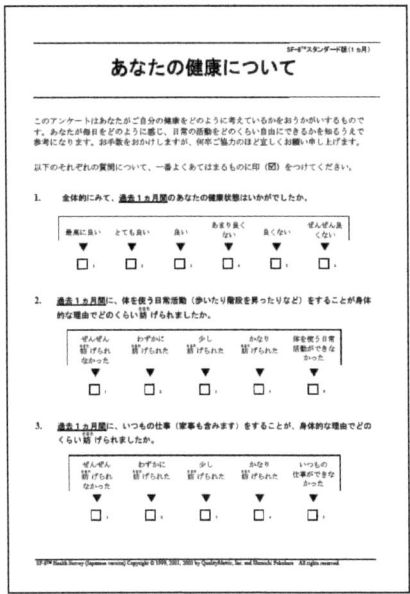

Figure 1: SF-8 Japanese version

7

3) Oral functions

The following 5 items were examined: risk of dysphagia, tongue pressure, force of lip closure, occlusal force, and articulatory function.

(1) Risk of dysphgia

The dysphagia risk assessment for community-dwelling elderly (DRACE, Figure 2)[17] is a questionnaire composed of 12 items that was developed to evaluate swallowing function deterioration in community-dwelling elderly people. The scale comprises the following questions: "do you sometimes have a fever?", "do you feel as though having a meal is more time-consuming than before?", "do you sometimes feel as though swallowing is difficult?", "do you sometimes feel as though it is difficult to eat something hard?", "does food sometimes spill out of your mouth?", "do you sometimes choke during your meals?", "do you sometimes choke when you drink liquid such as tea?", "are there times when the things you swallowed flow back into your nose?", "does your voice sometimes change after eating or drinking?", "does sputum form in your throat during meals or after eating or drinking?", "do you sometimes feel as though food gets stuck in your chest?", and "are there times when food or a sour fluid flows back from your stomach toward your throat?". The scale includes findings of dysphagia from the preparatory phase to the esophageal phase in a well-balanced manner. The likelihood of occurrence of each item was rated according to the following 3 levels ranging from 0 to 2: "occurs frequently: 0", "occurs sometimes: 1", and "never occurs: 2". The pulmonary dysphagia risk was determined according to the total score. An increase in the DRACE score shows an increased risk of swallowing function deterioration, and a score of 5 or higher suggests a risk of pulmonary dysphagia[18].

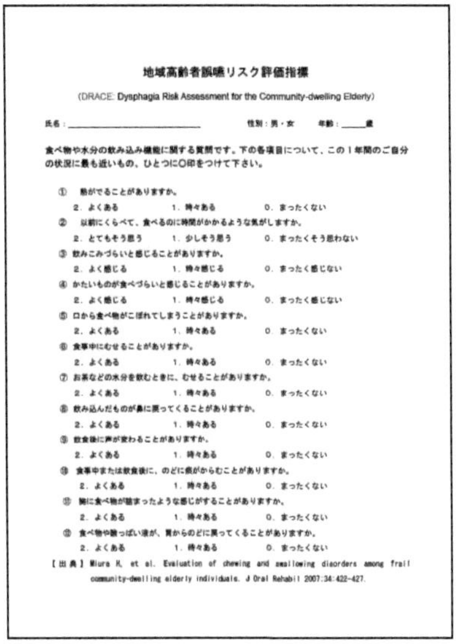

地域高齢者誤嚥リスク評価指標

(DRACE: Dysphagia Risk Assessment for the Community-dwelling Elderly)

氏名 : ＿＿＿＿＿＿＿＿＿＿＿＿＿＿ 性別 : 男・女 年齢 : ＿＿＿歳

食べ物や水分の飲み込み機能に関する質問です。下の各項目について、この1年間のご自分
の状況に最も近いもの、ひとつに○印をつけて下さい。

① 熱がでることがありますか。
　2. よくある　　　　1. 時々ある　　　　0. まったくない
② 以前にくらべて、食べるのに時間がかかるような気がしますか。
　2. とてもそう思う　　1. 少しそう思う　　0. まったくそう思わない
③ 飲みこみづらいと感じることがありますか。
　2. よく感じる　　　　1. 時々感じる　　　0. まったく感じない
④ かたいものが食べづらいと感じることがありますか。
　2. よく感じる　　　　1. 時々感じる　　　0. まったく感じない
⑤ 口から食べ物がこぼれてしまうことがありますか。
　2. よくある　　　　1. 時々ある　　　　0. まったくない
⑥ 食事中にむせることがありますか。
　2. よくある　　　　1. 時々ある　　　　0. まったくない
⑦ お茶などの水分を飲むときに、むせることがありますか。
　2. よくある　　　　1. 時々ある　　　　0. まったくない
⑧ 飲み込んだものが鼻に戻ってくることがありますか。
　2. よくある　　　　1. 時々ある　　　　0. まったくない
⑨ 飲食後に声が変わることがありますか。
　2. よくある　　　　1. 時々ある　　　　0. まったくない
⑩ 食事中または就寝前に、のどに痰がからむことがありますか。
　2. よくある　　　　1. 時々ある　　　　0. まったくない
⑪ 喉に食べ物が詰まったような感じがすることがありますか。
　2. よくある　　　　1. 時々ある　　　　0. まったくない
⑫ 食べ物や酸っぱい液が、胃からのどに戻ってくることがありますか。
　2. よくある　　　　1. 時々ある　　　　0. まったくない

【出典】Miura H, et al. Evaluation of chewing and swallowing disorders among frail
community-dwelling elderly individuals. J Oral Rehabil 2007;34:422-427.

Figure 2: The 12 questions of the DRACE

(2) Tongue pressure

TPM-01, a tongue pressure measuring instrument (manufactured by JMS Co., Ltd., Hiroshima, Japan, Figure 3), was used to measure tongue pressure. This tongue pressure measuring instrument comprises a digital tongue pressure meter, connecting tube, and tongue pressure probe. The balloon section of the tongue pressure probe, which was automatically pressurized as predetermined by the measurement device, was inserted onto the oral part of the tongue while the participant was seated; the participant was instructed to elevate the tip of the tongue to the palate at a maximum force for 5 to 7 seconds, during which the intensity of the force that crushed the balloon was measured. The tongue pressure measurement was performed twice consecutively in accordance with the method described in previous studies[19], and the mean of the measured values was recorded as the tongue pressure level (kPa). Elderly adults aged 70 years or older are considered to require a tongue pressure level of 20 kPa or greater[19].

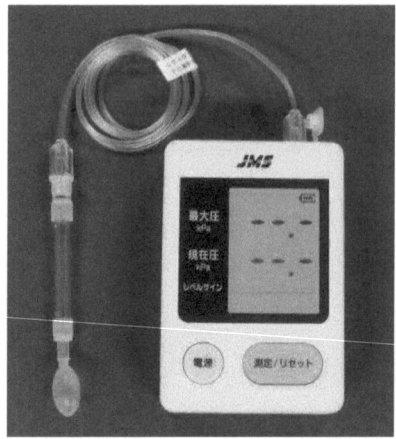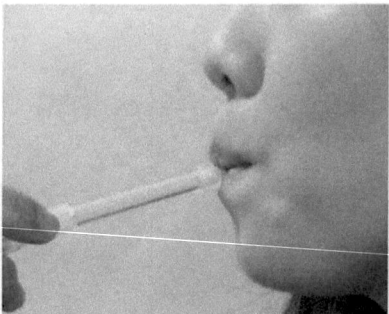

Figure 3: Tongue pressure measuring instrument

(3) Lip closure force

To measure the lip closure force, a lip force measuring instrument, Lip de Cum LDC-110® (manufactured by Cosmo Instruments Co., Ltd., Tokyo, Japan, **Figure 4**), was used. Lip de Cum® was used after attaching 2 of the supplied plastic Duckling® lip holders to the main unit. The Ducklings® were sandwiched between the upper and lower lips, and the maximum force required to close the lips was measured[20]. In this study, the force was measured twice consecutively, and the mean of the measured values was recorded as the intensity of lip closure force (N). A previous study showed that the intensities of the lip closure force among participants aged 80–84 years were 7.1 ± 5.3 N in men and 5.8 ± 2.6 N in women[20].

10

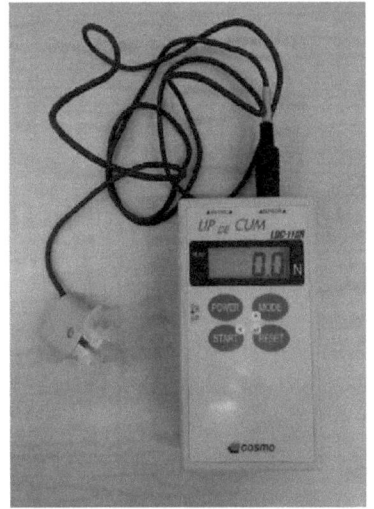
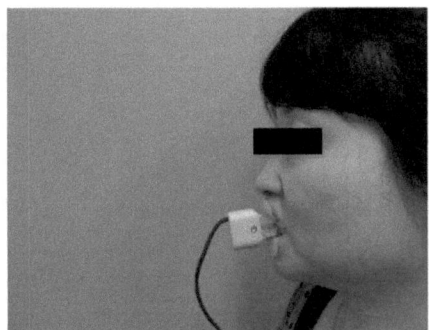

Figure 4: Lip de Cum

(4) Occlusal force

The occlusal force was measured with an occlusal force measurement system Occluser (FPD-707, manufactured by GC Dental Products Corporation, Tokyo, Japan, Figure 5). Dental Prescale, a film intended for exclusive use with this device, was fixed to the biting surfaces of the teeth, and the participants were instructed to bite by exerting force in 1 effort. The Pre-scale causes film development according to the intensity of the occlusal force, and setting the film in the Occluser cassette allows the data to be read. The data are converted into pressure values and displayed on a monitor.

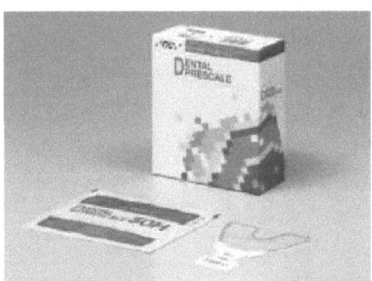

Figure 5: Dental Prescale

11

(5) Articulatory function

Oral diadochokinesis was used to evaluate the speed and regularity of articulatory organ movements through alternating repetitive movements by instructing the participants to pronounce syllables as rapidly as possible[21]. In this study, data were obtained by instructing the participants to repeatedly utter 3 syllables often used in the Japanese language, namely /pa/, /ta/, and /ka/, as well as a complex phrase consisting of these syllables in combination: /pataka/. The syllable /pa/ allowed the evaluation of lip functions, /ta/ allowed the evaluation of the functions of the anterior part of the tongue, and /ka/ allowed the evaluation of the functions of the posterior part of the tongue. The measurements were performed in a quiet space; the participants were instructed to perform the syllable articulation movements as fast as possible, and the resulting sounds were recorded for 5 seconds each on a recorder (LS-11, manufactured by Olympus Corporation, Tokyo, Japan). Waveforms corresponding to the syllables were extracted from the recorded audio data with acoustic analysis software, and the number of utterances per 5 seconds were counted, after which the values (number of utterances of the 3 syllables /pa/, /ta/, and /ka/) per 1 second were calculated. In addition, for the combined phrase composed of 3 syllables (/pataka/), the number of times uttered per 5 seconds was calculated as the number of syllables divided by 3.

4) Intra-oral environment

The following 3 items were examined: number of teeth, amount of saliva, and bacterial count in the oral cavity.

(1) Number of teeth

For subjects wearing a denture, the denture was removed and only the current number of teeth was counted.

(2) Amount of saliva

Saliva collection was performed by using Salikids tubes (manufactured by Sarstedt AG & Co., Nümbrecht, Germany), which were designed exclusively for saliva collection. A sponge used exclusively for saliva collection was placed under the tongue of a seated participant. While the participant rested, the sponge remained in place for 60 seconds and was subsequently removed. The weight of the saliva absorbed by the sponge was measured using an electronic balance (Adventurer Pro, manufactured by Ohaus Corporation, Parsippany, NJ, USA).

(3) Bacterial count in the oral cavity

The bacterial count (cfu/ml saliva) was measured using a bacterial counter (manufactured by Panasonic Corporation, Kadoma, Osaka, Japan, Figure 6). The upper surface of the tongue was wiped with a cotton swab included in the kit; the swab was subsequently inserted into a measurement sensor cup and the bacterial count was determined.The measurement results were rated digitally and categorized into 7 different levels. A higher level indicated an increased bacterial count. The median of the elderly person is level 4 (3.16×10^6 cfu/ml $\sim 1 \times 10^7$ cfu/ml).

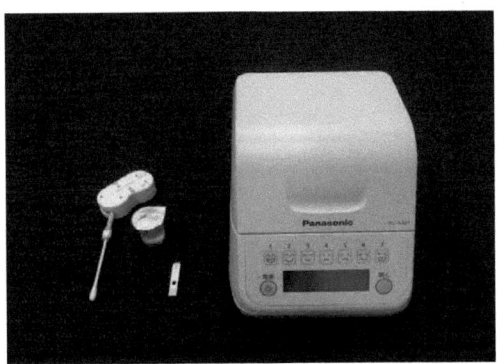

Figure 6: bacterial counter

5) Oral care status

The following were surveyed via questionnaire: oral cleaning frequency, history of dental consultation and the reason for consultation, awareness or non-awareness of oral functional exercises, the extent of oral functional exercise actually performed, and the performance or non-performance of site-specific oral functional exercises.

4. Analysis method

Associations with the oral cavity condition were analyzed using a bivariate analysis and multivariate analysis. The significance level was set at <0.05. The statistical software IBM SPSS Ver. 20.0 (SPSS, Inc., Chicago, IL, USA) was used for the statistical analyses.

13

5. Ethical considerations

This study was conducted after obtaining consent from the participants as well as from individuals affiliated with the surveyed facilities; the following were fully explained to the participants and affiliated individuals: the study purpose, procedure, optional nature of study participation, protection of personal information, and results publication.

In addition, the survey in this study was conducted after obtaining approval from the Research Ethics Review Committee of the School of Nursing at the University of KinDAI Himeji, following a review by the Research Ethics Review Board of the National Institute of Public Health.

III. Results

1. Basic attributes and oral health status

1) Basic attributes

(1) Age and sex

The participant age was 81.6 ± 7.4 years, and the participants comprised 86 men (38.2%) and 139 women (61.8%).

(2) ADL

The following scores were obtained using the ADL20 evaluation method: total score: 46.39 ± 10.18; basic ADL score: 26.96 ± 5.32; instrumental ADL score: 13.68 ± 5.63; and communication ADL score: 5.71 ± 0.80.

(3) Nutritional status

BMI

The BMI was 22.64 ± 3.98. In addition, the stature was 152.22 ± 10.00 cm, and the body weight was 52.80 ± 11.13 kg.

MNA-SF

The MNA-SF score was 10.09±2.57; 76 participants (35.8%) received scores of 12–14, indicating "good nutritional status", 99 (46.7%) received scores of 8–11, indicating "at risk of malnutrition", and 37 (17.5%) received scores of 0–7, indicating "malnutrition" (Figure 7).

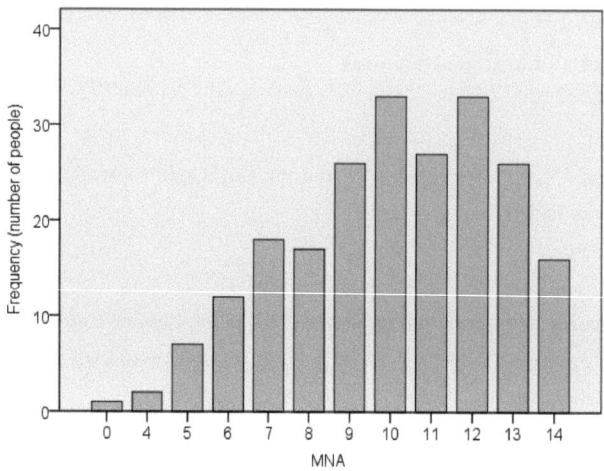

Figure 7: Distribution of MNA scores in community-dwelling dependent elderly persons

(4) Current disease

The following diseases affected the participants at the time of the survey and within the previous 1-year period: stroke: 41 participants (18.8%); rheumatism: 7 (3.2%); degenerative bone diseases: 31 (14.2%); bone fracture: 30 (13.8%); neuralgia: 19 (8.7%); Parkinson's disease: 9 (4.1%); hypertension: 76 (34.9%); heart disease: 28 (12.8%); diabetes: 33 (15.1%); kidney disease: 5 (2.3%); cancer: 11 (5.0%); pneumonia: 11 (5.0%); influenza: 7 (3.2%); dementia: 9 (4.1%); and psychiatric disorders (except dementia): 8 (3.7%).

2) Health-related QOL

The following mean scores were obtained in the SF-8 sub-areas: PF: 45.97 ± 7.55; RP: 45.54 ± 8.67; BP: 47.94 ± 9.39; GH: 47.80 ± 7.37; VT: 47.89 ± 6.91; SF: 45.20 ± 8.95; RE: 48.10 ± 7.67; and MH: 48.36 ± 7.22. All of these scores were lower than the national standard values (Table 1).

16

Table 1: SF-8 results in community-dwelling dependent elderly persons and comparison with national standard values

SF-8 sub-items	Dependent community-dwelling elderly persons	National standard values
PF (physical functioning)	45.97 ± 7.55	50.65 ± 5.22
RP (role-physical)	45.54 ± 8.67	51.42 ± 8.39
BP (bodily pain)	47.94 ± 9.39	50.99 ± 7.03
GH (general health perceptions)	47.80 ± 7.37	50.85 ± 4.79
VT (vitality)	47.89 ± 6.91	51.76 ± 6.02
SF (social functioning)	45.20 ± 8.95	50.09 ± 6.93
RE (role-emotional)	48.10 ± 7.67	50.96 ± 6.51
MH (mental health)	48.36 ± 7.22	50.89 ± 5.12

3) Oral functions

(1) Risk of dysphagia: DRACE

The DRACE score was 4.43 ± 3.83, and 96 participants (43.4%) had a score of 5 or higher (Figure 8).

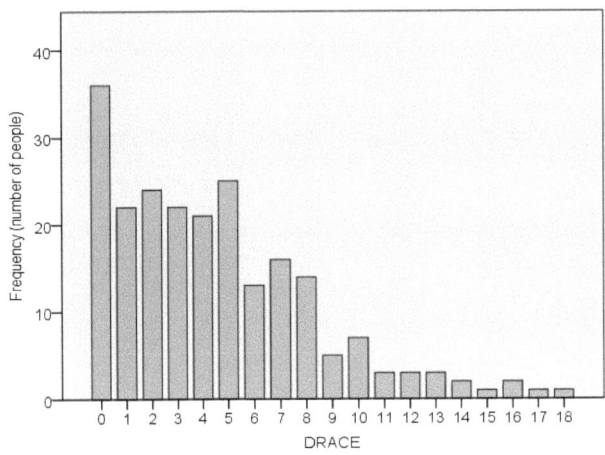

Figure 8: Distribution of DRACE scores in community-dwelling dependent elderly persons

(2) Tongue pressure

The tongue pressure was 23.96 ± 10.57 kPa. However, 64 participants (31.5%) did not achieve a force of 20 kPa, which is considered a standard value for those aged 70 years or older (Figure 9).

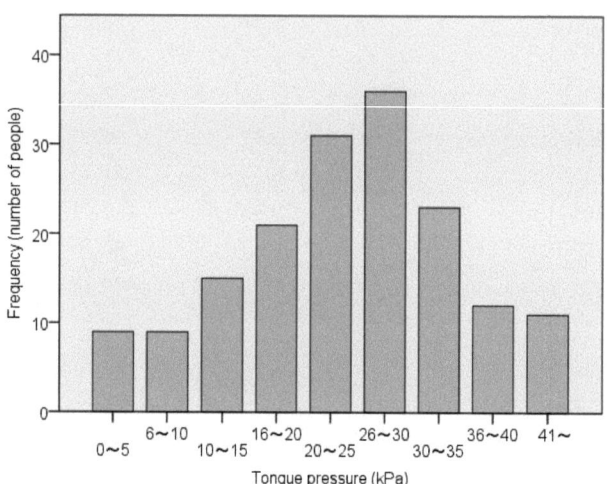

Figure 9: Tongue pressure distribution in community-dwelling dependent elderly persons

(3) Lip closure force

The lip closure force was 10.25 ± 5.99 N (Figure 10).

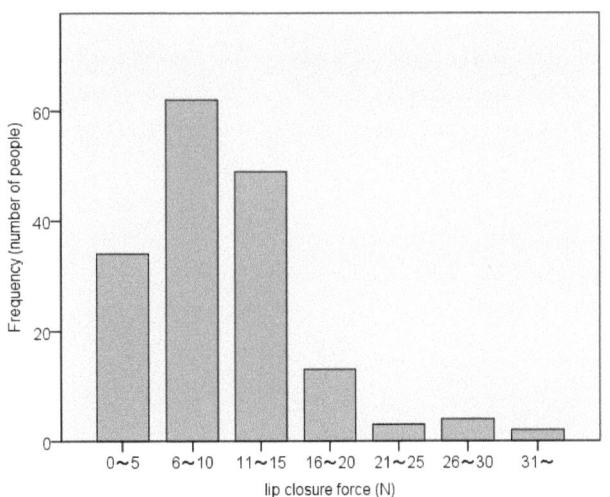

Figure 10: Distribution of lip closure force in among community-dwelling dependent elderly persons

(4) Occlusal force

The occlusal force was 492.65 ± 552.38 N (Figure 11).

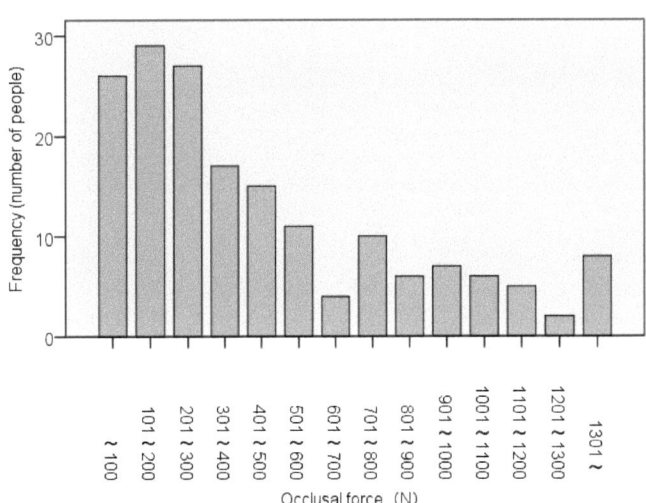

Figure 11: Occlusal force distribution in community-dwelling dependent elderly persons

19

(5) Articulatory function: oral diadochokinesis

The evaluated syllables were uttered as follows: /pa/: 4.93 ± 1.45 times; /ta/: 4.82 ± 1.37 times; and /ka/: 4.52 ± 1.31 times. The phrase /pataka/ was uttered 6.34 ± 3.29 times.

4) Intra-oral environment

(1) Number of teeth

The number of teeth was 11.33 ± 10.56, and 55 participants (26.6%) were edentulous (Figure 12).

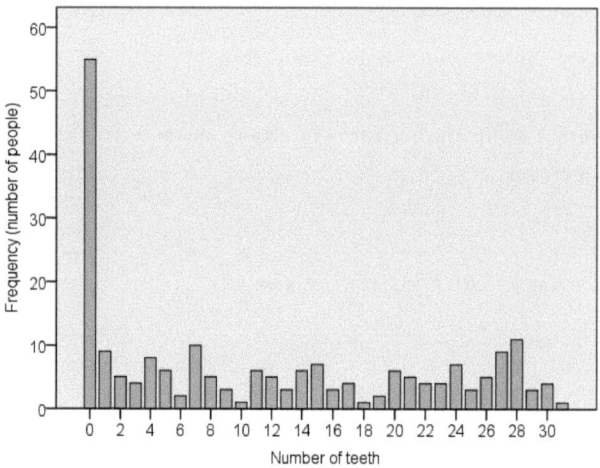

Figure 11: Number of teeth in community-dwelling dependent elderly persons

(2) Amount of saliva

The collected amount of saliva was 0.195 ± 0.210 mg.

(3) Bacterial count in the oral cavity

The bacterial levels were as follows: level 1: 4 participants (1.9%); level 2: 8 (3.9%); level 3: 27 (13.0%); level 4: 53 (25.6%); level 5: 85 (41.1%); level 6: 27 (13.0%); and level 7: 3 (1.4%). Overall, 115 participants (55.6%) were classified as level 5 or higher.

5) Oral care status

20

(1) Oral cleaning frequency

Forty-one participants (18.6%) "brushed their oral cavity 3 times or more per day", whereas 83 (37.7%), 82 (37.3%), 4 (1.8%), and 10 (4.6%) participants "brushed their oral cavity twice or more times per day", "brushed their oral cavity once or more per day", "brushed their oral cavity once every 2 or 3 days", and "almost never brushed their oral cavity" respectively.

(2) Degree of assistance needed for oral cleaning

Two hundred and eleven participants (95.4%) reported cleaning their mouths "without help", whereas 8 (3.6%) and 2 (0.9%) participants cleaned their mouths "with partial assistance or with someone to watch over them" and "with full-scale assistance", respectively.

(3) History of dental consultations and the major causes of dental consultations

Overall, 143 (65.3%) participants had "consulted dentists", whereas 76 (34.7%) had "virtually never consulted dentists". The major causes of dental consultations were as follows: treatment of dental caries: 45 participants (20.5%); gingival treatment: 21 (9.6%); cleaning of the teeth: 33 (15.1%); and adjustment of dentures: 78 (35.6%).

In addition, 3 participants (1.4%) had used visiting dental services.

(4) Awareness or non-awareness of oral functional exercises

Regarding awareness of oral functional exercises, 137 participants (62.8%) "knew about oral functional exercises" and 81 participants (37.2%) "did not know about oral functional exercises".

(5) Extent of oral functional exercises actually performed

In this category, 28 participants (12.9%) "performed oral functional exercises nearly every day", 93 (42.9%) "performed oral functional exercises every now and then", and 96 (44.2%) "never performed oral functional exercises".

(6) Performance or non-performance of site-specific oral functional exercises

The participants were asked whether they performed exercises, and those who responded as "having performed exercise" reported performing exercises related to the following 7 items: lip exercises: 72 participants (33.0%); tongue exercises: 95 (43.6%); practiced jaw exercises: 51 (23.4%); neck exercises, 67 (30.7%); exercises involving raising and lowering of shoulders: 73 (33.6%); exercises involving raising and lowering of arms: 62 (28.4%); and exercises involving word repetition: 79 (36.2%).

2. Associations with oral cavity conditions
1) Association between the oral cavity condition and health-related QOL
The association between the health-related QOL and the items for evaluating the oral cavity condition, specifically the 5 factors pertaining to oral functions and 3 factors pertaining to the intra-oral environment, was analyzed using a bivariate analysis (Pearson's and Spearman's correlation coefficients). DRACE differed significantly with respect to the SF-8 sub-area scores, with correlation coefficients of 0.3 or higher. Among the SF-8 sub-areas, GH, SF, RE, and MH were significantly associated with DRACE. The results demonstrated a slightly weak correlation, suggesting a possible association between DRACE and SF-8. Meanwhile, there were no associations with other items pertaining to the oral cavity condition (Table 2).

Table 2: Results of the bivariate analysis of DRACE and SF-8

SF-8 sub-areas	n	Correlation coefficient(r)	Significance probability (p)
PF (physical functioning)	218	-0.16	<0.02[*]
RP (role-physical)	218	-0.18	<0.01[**]
BP (bodily pain)	218	-0.19	<0.01[**]
GH (general health perceptions)	218	-0.35	<0.01[**]
VT (vitality)	219	-0.27	<0.01[**]
SF (social functioning)	219	-0.35	<0.01[**]
RE (role-emotional)	219	-0.32	<0.01[**]
MH (mental health)	219	-0.42	<0.01[**]

· Pearson's correlation coefficient

· [*]p <0.05, [**]p <0.01

Regarding DRACE, which exhibited a significant association with SF-8 in the bivariate analyses, a stepwise multiple regression analysis was performed to eliminate the influences of confounding factors. Analyses were conducted in which DRACE was set as a dependent variable and typical confounding factors (age, sex,

22

and level of care needed) were added to the 8 sub-areas of SF-8 as input variables. In multiple regression analyses, 2 of the SF-8 sub-areas, namely GH and MH, exhibited significant differences (Table 3).

Table 3: Results of the multiple regression analysis of DRACE and SF-8 (N = 218)

Variable	Standardized coefficient (β)	t value	Significance probability (p)
MH	-0.33	-4.57	<0.01 [**]
SF	-0.17	-2.27	<0.05 [*]

· Stepwise multiple regression analysis: R = 0.44, R^2 = 0.20, adjusted R^2 = 0.19
· Dependent variable: DRACE
· Input variables: age, sex, level of care required, SF-8 sub-areas (PF, RP, BP, GH, VT, SF, RE, MH)

2) Association between the oral cavity condition and nutritional status

The associations of MNA-SF with the 5 oral function items and 3 intra-oral environment items were analyzed using a bivariate analysis (Spearman and Spearman's correlation coefficient). DRACE differed significantly with respect to MNA-SF, with correlation coefficients of 0.3 or higher. The results demonstrated a slightly weak correlation, suggesting a possible association between DRACE and MNA-SF. Meanwhile, there were no associations with the other items pertaining to the oral cavity condition (Table 4).

Table 4: Results of the bivariate analysis of oral functions and MNA

Oral functions	n	Correlation coefficient (r)	Significance probability (p)
Risk of dysphagia (DRACE)	218	-0.36	<0.01**
Tongue pressure	197	0.17	<0.02*
Force of lip closure	197	0.25	<0.01**
Occlusal force	170	0.05	0.48
OD /pa/	191	-0.04	0.60
OD /ta/	190	0.07	0.36
OD /ka/	188	0.12	0.10
OD /pataka/	188	0.17	<0.02*

- Pearson's correlation coefficient
- *$p < 0.05$, **$p < 0.01$
- OD: oral diadochokinesis

Regarding DRACE, which exhibited a significant association with MNA-SF in the bivariate analyses, a stepwise multiple regression analysis was performed to eliminate the influences of confounding factors. Analyses were conducted in which DRACE was set as a dependent variable and typical confounding factors (age, sex, and level of care needed) were added to MNA as input variables. Similar to the correlation coefficient, DRACE exhibited a significant association with MNA (Table 5).

Table 5: Results of the multiple regression analysis of DRACE and MNA (N = 217)

Variable	Standardized coefficient (β)	t value	Significance probability (p)
MNA	-.34	-5.36	<0.01**

- Stepwise multiple regression analysis: $R = 0.34$, $R^2 = 0.12$, Adjusted $R^2 = 0.11$
- Dependent variable: DRACE
- Input variables: age, sex, level of care needed, MNA
- **$p < 0.01$

3) Association between oral functions and the performance or non-performance of site-specific oral functional exercises

The associations between the 5 oral function items and 7 oral functional exercise items were analyzed using a t-test.

Articulatory function differed significantly with respect to the performance or non-performance of lip exercises. The number of utterances of the oral diadochokinesis /ka/ was significantly higher among elderly subjects who practiced lip exercises than among those who did not (Table 6).

Table 6: Results of an analysis of the association between oral functions and lip exercises

Oral functions	Mean ± SD (n)		p-value
	Subjects who performed exercises	Subjects who did not perform exercises	
DRACE	4.32 ± 3.56 (72)	4.48 ± 3.97 (146)	0.77
Tongue pressure (kPa)	24.68 ± 8.96 (66)	23.60 ± 11.31 (131)	0.47
Lip closure (N)	11.19 ± 6.09 (66)	9.70 ± 5.94 (131)	0.10
Occlusal force (N)	508.72 ± 698.10 (60)	486.41 ± 462.85 (110)	0.80
OD /pa/	5.17 ± 1.45 (63)	4.81 ± 1.45 (128)	0.11
OD /ta/	4.99 ± 1.36 (63)	4.71 ± 1.39 (127)	0.18
OD /ka/	4.89 ± 1.18 (61)	4.34 ± 1.34 (127)	<0.01 [**]
OD /pataka/	7.03 ± 3.07 (61)	6.10 ± 4.03 (127)	0.11

· t-test

· [**]p <0.01

· OD: oral diadochokinesis, SD: standard deviation

Articulatory function differed significantly with respect to the performance or non-performance of tongue exercises. Compared to elderly subjects who did not practice tongue exercises, those who practiced the exercises uttered significantly higher numbers of the oral diadochokinesis sounds /pa/, /ka/ and /pataka/ (Table 7).

Table 7 : Results of an analysis of the association between oral functions and tongue exercises

Oral functions	Mean ± SD (n)		p-value
	Subjects who performed exercises	Subjects who did not perform exercises	
DRACE	4.23 ± 3.46 (95)	4.58 ± 4.10 (123)	0.50
Tongue pressure (kPa)	25.21 ± 9.71 (88)	23.00 ± 11.17 (109)	0.14
Lip closure force (N)	10.71 ± 5.59 (87)	9.80 ± 6.33 (110)	0.30
Occlusal force (N)	472.89 ± 360.42 (81)	513.76 ± 688.06 (89)	0.63
OD /pa/	5.18 ± 1.54 (83)	4.73 ± 1.36 (108)	<0.04 [*]
OD /ta/	4.98 ± 1.45 (83)	4.66 ± 1.32 (107)	0.12
OD /ka/	4.82 ± 1.32 (82)	4.28 ± 1.26 (106)	<0.01 [**]
OD /pataka/	7.11 ± 3.30 (82)	5.86 ± 4.02 (106)	<0.03 [*]

· t-test

· [*] $p < 0.05$, [**] $p < 0.01$

· OD: oral diadochokinesis, SD: standard deviation

The lip closure force differed significantly depending on the performance or non-performance of shoulder raising and lowering exercises. Elderly subjects who performed shoulder raising and lowering exercises had a significantly stronger lip closure force than those who did not perform such exercises (Table 8).

Table 8: Results of an analysis of the association between oral functions and shoulder raising and lowering exercises

Oral functions	Mean ± SD (n)		p-value
	Subjects who performed exercises	Subjects who did not perform exercises	
DRACE	4.45 ± 3.72 (73)	4.40 ± 3.91 (144)	0.92
Tongue pressure (kPa)	24.93 ± 9.98 (70)	23.43 ± 10.89 (127)	0.34
Lip closure force (N)	11.39 ± 6.83 (70)	9.54 ± 5.43 (127)	<0.04*
Occlusal force (N)	503.56 ± 697.05 (63)	488.82 ± 455.48 (107)	0.87
OD /pa/	4.86 ± 1.56 (66)	4.96 ± 1.41 (125)	0.65
OD /ta/	4.67 ± 1.51 (66)	4.87 ± 1.31 (124)	0.35
OD /ka/	4.54 ± 1.37 (65)	4.51 ± 1.29 (123)	0.85
OD /pataka/	7.03 ± 4.57 (65)	6.07 ± 3.22 (123)	0.10

· t-test

· *p <0.05

· OD: oral diadochokinesis, SD: standard deviation

The swallowing and articulatory functions differed significantly with respect to the performance or non-performance of word repetition exercises. Compared to elderly subjects who did not practice word repetition exercises, those who practiced such exercises exhibited a higher risk of dysphagia level as well as significantly more numerous utterances of the oral diadochokinesis sounds /pa/, /ka/, and /pataka/ (Table 9).

Table 9: Results of an analysis of the associations between oral functions and word repetition exercises

Oral functions	Mean ± SD (n)		p-value
	Subjects who performed exercises	Subjects who did not perform exercises	
DRACE	3.68 ± 2.69 (79)	4.85 ± 4.30 (139)	<0.02*
Tongue pressure (kPa)	24.45 ± 9.79 (77)	23.64 ± 11.07 (120)	0.60
Lip closure (N)	10.54 ± 4.65 (76)	9.99 ± 6.74 (121)	0.53
Occlusal force (N)	458.92 ± 374.30 (71)	519.65 ± 655.94 (99)	0.48
OD /pa/	5.19 ± 1.48 (73)	4.76 ± 1.43 (118)	<0.05*
OD /ta/	5.01 ± 1.37 (73)	4.67 ± 1.38 (117)	0.10
OD /ka/	4.89 ± 1.25 (72)	4.29 ± 1.30 (116)	<0.01**
OD /pataka/	7.65 ± 4.38 (72)	5.63 ± 3.09 (116)	<0.01**

· t-test

· *$p < 0.05$, **$p < 0.01$

· OD: oral diadochokinesis, SD: standard deviation

IV. Discussion

1. Oral health status among community-dwelling dependent elderly persons
1) Current oral function status

As the importance of oral functions in elderly people has been revealed, various methods have been developed to evaluate these functions. In the present study, a survey was conducted using multiple evaluation methods, and the results have elucidated the current status of oral functions in **community-dwelling dependent elderly persons** in Japan.

Methods for evaluating the swallowing function include the water-drinking test[22], which consists of actually swallowing liquids and foods, as well as the repetitive saliva swallowing test[23]; however, as the present study included subjects with some impairments, both safety and difficulty were considered; therefore, the evaluations were conducted via a questionnaire method in which the participants were instructed to answer questions regarding the presence or absence of symptoms related to swallowing function. The findings showed that most elderly subjects receiving long-term home care in Japan had symptoms of swallowing function deterioration. The participants in this study were elderly subjects requiring nursing care, but for most the extent of care needed was relatively low; nonetheless, the percentage of participants with a DRACE score of 5 or greater was as high as 43.4%, indicating a risk of dysphagia, and this may be a major issue from the perspective of elder care. In addition, the mean DRACE score among the surveyed participants was 4.43 ± 3.83, which was elevated considerably relative to the DRACE value (3.47 ± 3.32) reported in a survey[24] of independent elderly subjects in the same age group, suggesting a potentially higher pulmonary dysphagia risk among elderly subjects requiring nursing care relative to independent elderly subjects. The findings suggested that a risk of dysphagia was present in a considerable number of **community-dwelling dependent elderly persons** and that in the future, home care interventions that account for swallowing function deterioration will be in high demand.

Approximately 30% of the participants in this study failed to achieve a tongue pressure of 20 kPa (standard pressure for individuals aged 70 years or older). The tongue pressure is a necessary force to send the alimentary bolus into the pharynx during deglutition, and reports from previous studies have shown that among elderly subjects, tongue pressure is associated with the masticatory function[25] and dietary patterns[26]; therefore, tongue pressure may be a key element that influences food intake and swallowing. Reports based on studies of elderly individuals in geriatric health service facilities have indicated tongue pressures of 19.2 ± 8.1 kPa[27] and 15.22 ± 9.14 kPa[28]; however, the mean value of 23.96 ± 10.57 kPa found among our study participants was higher than that found among the institutionalized elderly subjects in the earlier reports. In addition, in a survey of independent elderly subjects [19], the tongue pressure was found to be 31.9 ± 8.9 kPa, a higher value than that reported in our study. In elderly subjects, tongue pressure has also been indicated to associate with ADL[26)29)], and therefore, the differences in tongue pressure values observed in the surveyed elderly subjects might have been due to the influence of differences in ADL. For most **community-dwelling dependent elderly persons**, the level of care needed is lower than that of elderly subjects institutionalized in geriatric health service facilities, and the extent of ADL may have an impact on tongue pressure.

A comparison of the mean lip closure force observed in our study participants (10.25 ± 5.99 N) with measured values obtained using the same measurement devices as those used in our study revealed that the values in our study were higher than those reported for male (4.9 ± 8.0 N) and female (4.8 ± 8.3 N) elderly individuals institutionalized in geriatric health service facilities[29] and were similar to the value reported for independent elderly subjects (10.9 ± 3.6 N)[30]. In addition, the lip function reserve capacity has been shown to be reduced in elderly subjects relative to younger adults[31]; however, in another report the lip closure force was not associated with age[26)32)]. Our survey data showed no association between the lip closure force and age. The number of reported epidemiological studies of tongue pressure and lip closure force in elderly subjects is small, and the measured values can differ depending on the measurement method. However, in recent years associations have been reported between the tongue pressure and nutritional status[9], as well as between lip-closing movements and brain activity[33)34)]. These findings suggest that the tongue pressure and lip closure force might also influence the general health of elderly subjects. Therefore, research in the area of geriatric oral health, using tongue pressure and lip closure force as evaluation indices, should be promoted as this may contribute to the development of elderly care in the future.

The occlusal force is influenced by the number of teeth, and values of 432.7 ± 214.6 N and 438.9 ± 310.2 N have been reported in independent elderly subjects[35], as well as values of 502.4 N in male and 372.2 N in female individuals[36]; this suggests that the occlusal force values obtained in our study were similar to those observed previously in independent elderly subjects. In addition, sex differences in the occlusal force have been reported[36)37)] and in our study, the values were found to be significantly higher in men than in women. In addition, the occlusal force has been reported to decrease markedly in individuals aged 80 years or older, and the following have been reported as associated factors: physical strength, mobility, and lifestyle habits[36)]. However, few reports have addressed the occlusal force in elderly subjects, and an accumulation of data and study of standard values may be needed in the future.

Oral diadochokinesis was used in this study to evaluate the articulatory function. In a previous study of frail elderly subjects, the reported mean oral diadochokinesis values were as follows: /pa/ was uttered 4.9 times per second, /ta/ was uttered 4.8 times per second, and /ka/was uttered 4.5 times per second[38)]. These values were the same as those obtained in our study. Although both the previously reported frail elderly people and the **community-dwelling dependent elderly persons** in our study required some assistance, their physical and psychological conditions allowed them to participate in daily activities to some extent. Therefore, the articulatory functions of frail elderly subjects and those requiring mild nursing care might be very similar. The articulatory function is said to deteriorate with aging and with a decrease in ADL[38)]; however, in the presence of a functional decline in the elderly, assistance consistent with the extent of the function is considered necessary. Oral diadochokinesis reference values, for which research studies are ongoing[39)], are needed in the daily lives of elderly individuals. A target level of articulatory function is needed, along with examinations of the subjects' physical and psychological conditions and interventions adapted to their needs.

The previously described findings, which include our study results, suggest that despite some differences in each of the oral function evaluation items, dependent community-dwelling elderly persons exhibited oral function values between those of institutionalized elderly subjects and of independent elderly subjects. In addition, the findings also suggested that the need for assistance consequent to oral function deterioration might also account for the extremely high percentage of **community-dwelling dependent elderly persons**. To meet these needs, a system must be constructed to allow **community-dwelling dependent elderly persons** to have an accurate understanding of their own oral function condition and to receive proper care from a professional when necessary. For an accurate understanding of the oral function condition in elderly subjects, regular professional evaluation would be preferable; however, unlike institutionalized elderly subjects who live in groups, elderly individuals living at home are scattered in individual residences and for that reason, it is difficult to set up a time and place for oral function evaluation. Therefore, screening methods that could be easily used by the elderly themselves or their close family members need to be developed and disseminated. The DRACE, which was used in this study, allows evaluation of the swallowing function based on the responses to 12 items and as a result is less burdensome and can be used easily; therefore, this tool it could be utilized in evaluations of **community-dwelling dependent elderly persons**. Meanwhile, using the tongue pressure and lip closure force as evaluation items would be burdensome because of the specialized equipment required for the measurements. In **community-dwelling dependent elderly persons**, the ability to reach the corners of the mouth with the tip of the tongue has been found to associate significantly with the tongue pressure and lip closure force[40], and therefore the numerical value obtained by measuring the speed of this motion could be used as a simple evaluation index and alternative to measuring the tongue pressure and lip closure force.

2) Current intra-oral environment status

In 2011, a nationwide survey conducted in Japan revealed that the percentage of "elderly 8020 achievers" (i.e., the percentage of people with 20 or more natural teeth at the age of 80 years) was 38.3%, a considerable increase in comparison with the 24.1% reported in 2005. In surveyed elderly subjects aged 80 to 84 years, the reported number of teeth was 12.2, similar to the findings of the present study, in which the reported number of teeth was 11.33. This difference might be due to the effect of the "8020 movement", which has been proposed in Japan since the year 1989. The "8020 movement", which was implemented in Japan to prevent tooth loss in the elderly, may need to be disseminated worldwide.

Reportedly, the amount of saliva secretion ranges from 1000 to 1500 ml per day (0.7 to 1.0 ml per minute), and whereas some reports have stated that salivary secretion is not affected by sex or age[41][42], it is believed to be reduced in most elderly individuals as a result of the influence of the medications taken to treat the increasingly prevalent diseases associated with old age[43]. In our study, the collected amount of saliva was approximately 0.2 mg per minute, and the participants tended to have dry oral cavities. Although previous reports have shown an association between the amount of saliva and the *Candida albicans* cell count in the oral cavity[44], saliva is known to exhibit antimicrobial activity, and a decrease in the amount of saliva inhibits bacterial suppression in the oral cavity, increasing

32

the risk intra-oral environmental deterioration.

In this study, a bacterial counter was used to measure the bacterial cell counts; in previous studies of elderly subjects that used the same type of device, the median value was 4 and 55% of subjects had a value of 5 or higher, indicating bacterial cell counts of at least 10 million. Similarly, in previous studies[45)46)], the presence of bacteria within the oral cavity has been reported in a high percentage of elderly subjects requiring nursing care, and trends similar to those found in our study have been shown. Our study also suggested that the presence of high levels of bacteria in the oral cavity was a contributing factor to the development of pneumonia and endocarditis in community-dwelling dependent elderly persons and was also a critical issue that affected the vital prognosis. The findings suggest a strong need for assistance in dealing with the presence of bacteria in the oral cavity in terms of intra-oral environment maintenance in community-dwelling dependent elderly persons.

3) Current oral care status

In this study, the oral hygiene status was examined as organic oral care. The resulting data showed that a large number of elderly individuals performed oral cleaning on a daily basis, and more than 95% of elderly people performed oral cleaning by themselves, without any help. In addition, few individuals (1.4%) received dental care through home visits; on the other hand, among those who consulted dental offices, a higher percentage did so for the purpose of adjusting their dentures versus oral care. The results showed that for dependent community-dwelling elderly persons, oral cleaning has become a daily lifestyle habit and that even when these subjects were in situations requiring some form of nursing care, they rarely received nursing assistance with oral cleaning. In preventive nursing care projects conducted in Japan, elderly individuals with physical function deterioration had a certain sense of participation in preventive nursing care projects, whereas among elderly individuals with oral function deterioration, the rate of participation in preventive nursing care projects was extremely low. Elderly people are less likely to be aware of the need for oral cavity care and as a result, oral cavity prevention and care is at risk of being taken lightly and considered by the elderly as something they can perform sufficiently by themselves, without any assistance.

Oral cleaning is primarily performed to remove residues and bacteria inside the oral cavity; however, the participants in our study exhibited high levels of bacteria in their oral cavities, suggesting that their cleanings were not sufficiently effective. Therefore, routine mouth cleaning alone, which is performed as a daily lifestyle habit, may not be sufficient to reduce the amount of bacteria in the oral cavity. In a study[47] of thorough professional oral health care conducted by dentists and dental hygienists in community-dwelling dependent elderly persons, the findings showed that oral cleaning for 1 to 2 months had no reducing effect on the bacterial counts in the pharynx, and a significant decrease in bacterial count was observed only after 5 months of intervention. In addition, morbidity due to pneumonia has been reported to decrease after an intervention of up to 24 months' duration[48]. This suggests that oral cleaning performed by the elderly themselves, as well as short-term interventions, had an extremely localized effect in the reduction of oral bacteria. However, specialized oral care performed by dental professionals led to a significant decrease in the incidence of dysphagia pneumonia[48] and improved the intra-oral environment. To reduce the risks due to oral bacteria, the professional expertise of dentists and dental hygienists should be put into practice continually and the elderly individuals themselves, or close family members who act as caregivers, may need to become acquainted with the skills thereof. The current system of daily oral cleaning performed by the elderly themselves requires revision, and in order to improve the bacterial levels in the intra-oral environment, measures to increase quality of organic oral care may need to be examined.

In recent years, various oral functional exercise techniques have been promoted as a means of maintaining and improving oral functions. Therefore, in our study, oral functional exercises were performed as functional oral care; however, approximately 40% of the elderly participants were unaware of these oral functional exercises, a finding that demonstrates the poor awareness of oral functional exercises. The findings suggest that for elderly people, the oral functions of ingestion and swallowing affect the vital prognosis, and thus awareness of the importance of care to prevent oral function deterioration should be increased.

2. Association between oral functions and health-related QOL

Eating is among the activities enjoyed by elderly people in their daily lives. In addition, the ingestion and swallowing functions have also been found to associate with the health-related QOL[49]; therefore, improving the functions of the oral cavity, an important food intake organ, is thought to lead to an improved QOL in elderly people.The bivariate analysis showed slightly weak correlations between the dysphagia risk and 4 of the 8 sub-areas of SF-8, suggesting that deterioration of the

34

swallowing function may lead to deterioration of the health-related QOL.

In addition, the results of multiple regression analyses after adjusting for confounding factors suggested a close association between the dysphagia risk and health-related QOL. The participants in this study had a mean age of 81.6 years, including a high percentage of older elderly subjects, and the daily life QOL might have been the most important element for those elderly individuals. Our study has revealed an association between the swallowing function and the QOL that further suggests the importance of interventions aimed at maintaining or improving oral functions, and particular focus on the swallowing function may be necessary.

In addition, in the elderly, oral function assessments are usually performed as interventions aimed at improving physical functioning and are mainly based on the results of an evaluation of physical functioning[50)51)]. Moreover, several reports[52) 53)] have shown that in elderly subjects who require nursing care and exhibit a considerable decline in basic ADL, the swallowing function was associated with physical health; therefore, in elderly subjects with a strong requirement for long-term nursing care, the swallowing function presumably has a particularly strong link with physical health-associated factors. However, it was extremely interesting that among the **community-dwelling dependent elderly persons** in our study, the swallowing function was closely associated with mental health QOL items such as SF and MH, but not with QOL items involving strong physical elements. Among elderly subjects requiring nursing care, those with a relatively low need for nursing care accounted for a high percentage among **community-dwelling dependent elderly persons**; in a survey of independent elderly subjects[9)], the swallowing function was reported to associate significantly with MH, and the effect of the swallowing function on health-related QOL varied depending on the level of care required by the elderly subjects and their home environments. For this reason, changes in the mental health-related QOL as an element of the outcome evaluation should possibly be considered when conducting an intervention aimed at improving the swallowing function in **community-dwelling dependent elderly persons**.

Our study findings suggest that the dysphagia risk might affect the health-related QOL; however, the associations between oral functions and physical aspects were also considerable. For the elderly subjects receiving long-term home care in our study, the MNA-SF evaluation demonstrated that after combining "those at risk of malnutrition" and "those with malnutrition", 65.1% of subjects faced problematic nutritional status issues; however, the MNA-SF of the participants was significantly associated with DRACE. This suggests that deterioration of the swallowing function might influence the nutritional status. A previous study demonstrated an association between the swallowing function and the MNA-SF in hospitalized elderly subjects[54]; in addition, a previous survey of institutionalized elderly subjects requiring nursing care revealed an association between tongue pressure and protein-energy malnutrition (PEM)[6]. Therefore, the oral functions might strongly affect the nutritional statuses of elderly subjects with diseases and disorders. To maintain the elderly subjects' overall health, interventions aimed at maintaining and improving the oral functions may lead to a reduced risk of malnutrition. Meanwhile, in the multiple regression analysis conducted in this study, the coefficient of determination was low, indicating a considerable influence of factors other than the oral functions. A previous study involving independent elderly subjects[30] showed a weak correlation between the current number of teeth, the current number of teeth supporting dental occlusion, and the albumin levels used for the numerical nutritional status evaluation; however, no significant association was found between the albumin levels and the results of a repetitive saliva swallowing test used for the numerical swallowing function evaluation. In addition, a previous report[55] described a correlation between MNA-SF and albumin levels in elderly subjects; however, another report[56] indicated that the majority of subjects would be classified as suffering from malnutrition according to MNA-SF evaluations of elderly individuals in Japan. It is currently impossible to determine whether the problematic issues and differences between the values were due to differences in the personal situations faced by the surveyed participants or differences in the methods used to evaluate the nutritional status; however, in dependent community-dwelling elderly persons, oral functioning is likely associated with the risk of malnutrition. The findings of our study reaffirmed the need to ensure oral function maintenance and improvement as a means of reducing the risk of malnutrition in addition to maintaining the QOL.

A previous study[57] reported oral functions improved in response to the performance of oral function improvement programs and oral care aimed at maintaining and improving oral functions. Because the swallowing function is associated with the health-related QOL, such approaches might not only lead to improved oral functions, but also to potentially considerable improvements in the QOL. Therefore, to improve the QOL, methods of delivering care that more effectively maintains and improves the oral functions are urgently needed. In our study, we surveyed the status of performing of oral functional exercises representative of functional oral care and analyzed their associations with oral functions. The findings suggest that among the oral functional exercises, lip exercises, tongue exercises, shoulder raising and lowering, and word repetition affected the articulatory function, swallowing function, and lip closure force. Oral functional exercises are believed to have beneficial effects on oral function maintenance and improvement, a belief that is supported by our study results. In addition, given the differences between the results, which depended on the type of oral functional exercise, specific exercises have been suggested to be more effective for specific oral functions. Although an elucidation of the details of these oral functional exercises will be a challenge in the future, given the fact that oral care is performed in busy work environments and in clinical settings, the development of effective intervention methods specialized for each segment and each function (e.g., swallowing) may be needed in addition to functional oral care, which is important for all oral functions.

V. Conclusions

This study revealed the following in regard to the current status of community-dwelling dependent elderly persons in Japan.

1. The subjects with the DRACE scores more than 5 to mean the high risk of dysphagia was 43.4%. 55.6% of subjects had a value of 5 or higher, indicating bacterial cell counts of at least 10 million. There was a considerable need for assistance with oral functions and the intra-oral environment.

2. Although 95% of the surveyed participants performed daily oral cleaning, only 13% performed daily oral functional exercises.

3. The dysphagia risk was associated with the health-related QOL and particularly affected the degree of psychological health, including social functioning and mental health.

4. The dysphagia risk was associated with the nutritional status.

5. Specific oral functions were associated with specific oral functional exercises.

Acknowledgments

The authors would like to express their heartfelt gratitude to all personnel involved with the daycare service facilities that collaborated in this study, as well as the senior citizens receiving long-term home care who participated in the surveys. This study was funded by a Grant-in-Aid for Scientific Research/Basic Research (C) [No.25463599] from the Japan Society for the Promotion of Science.

References

1) Kikuchi R, Watabe N, Konno T, Mishina N, Sekizawa K, Sasaki H: High incidence of silent dysphagia in elderly patients with community-acquired pneumonia. American Journal of Respiratory and Critical Care Medicine 1994; 150:251-253.

2) Itoh H, Kikutani T, Tamura F, Hamura A: The occlusal condition, feeding function and nutritional status of the dependent elderly at home. Japan Journal of Gerodontology 2008; 23:21-30.

3) Fukuoka Y, Hatakeyama R, Hatakeyama A, Sato A, Sasaki H: Oral care and dysphagia pneumonia. Antibiotics & Chemotherapy 2006; 22:602-606.

4) Yamawaki M: Epidemiology of dysphagia pneumonia. Sogo Rihabiriteshon 2009; 37:105-109.

5) Kasuya M: (5) Low nutrient condition malnutrition · High nutrient condition. Japanese Journal of Geriatrics 2013; 50:187-190.

6) Kodama M, Kikutani T, Yoshida M, Inaba S: Relationship between tongue pressure and malnutrition in the institutionalized elderly. Japan Journal of Gerodontology 2004; 19:161-167.

7) Morisaki N, Miura H: Analysis of risk factors related to dysphagia among disabled elderly individuals in geriatric health service facilities. Health Sciences 2010; 26:201-209.

8) Teraoka K, Morino T: Relationship between the vitality index and the oral function of the dependent elderly at a care facility. Japan Journal of Gerodontology 2009; 24:28-36.

9) Miura H, Hara S, Yamasaki K, Usui Y: Relationship between chewing and swallowing functions and health-related quality of life among elderly. Oral Health Care—Prosthodontics, Periodontology, Biology, Research and Systemic Conditions 2012;1-12.

10) Folstein MF, Folstein SE, McHugh PR: "Mini-mental state": A practical method for grading the cognitive state of patients for the clinician. Journal of Psychiatric Research 1975; 12:189-198.

11) Katoh S, Shimogaki H, Onodera A, Ueda H, Oikawa K, Ikeda K, et al.: Development of the revised version of Hasegawa's dementia scale (HDS-R). Japanese Journal of Geriatric Psychiatry 1991; 2:1339-1347.

12) Kahn RL, Goldfarb AI, Pollack M: Brief objective measures for the

determination of mental status in the aged. American Journal of Physiology 1960;117:326-328.

13)Eto F, Tanaka M, Chishima M, Igarashi M, Mizoguchi T, Wada H, et al.: Comprehensive activities of daily living (ADL) index for the elderly. Japanese Journal of Geriatrics 1992; 29:841-848.

14)Rubenstein LZ, Harker JO, Salva A, Guigoz Y, Vellas B: Screening for undernutrition in geriatric practice: Developing the short-form mini nutritional assessment (MNA-SF). The Journal of Gerontology 2001; 56A:366-377.

15)Vellas B, Villare H, Abellan G, Soto ME, Rolland Y, Guigoz Y, et al.: Overview of the MNA-Its history and challenges. The Journal of Nutrition, Health & Aging 2006;10:456-465.

16)Fukuhara S, Suzukamo Y: Instruments for measuring health-related quality of life —SF-8 and SF-36—.Journal of Clinical and Experimental Medicine 2005 ;213:133-136.

17)Miura H, Kariyasu M, Yamasaki K, Arai Y: Evaluation of chewing and swallowing disorders among frail community-dwelling elderly individuals. Journal of Oral Rehabilitation 2007; 34:422-427.

18)Takeuchi K, Aida J, Ito K, Furuta M, Yamashita Y, Osaka K: Nutritional status and dysphagia risk among community-dwelling frail older adults. Journal of Nutrition 2014; 18:352-357.

19)Utanohara Y, Hayashi R, Yoshikawa M, Yoshida M, Tsuga K, Akagawa Y: Standard values of maximum tongue pressure taken using newly developed disposable tongue pressure measurement device. Dysphagia 2008; 23:286-290.

20)Noro A, Hosokawa S, Takahashi J, Akihiro Y, Nishimoto Y, Hosokawa I, et al.: Basic and clinical changes of labial closure strength from youth to adults. The Japan Society of Conservative Dentistry 2002; 45:817-828.

21)Nishio M, Niimi S: A study on oral diadochokinesis in dysarthric speakers. The Japan Journal of Logopedics and Phoniatrics 2002; 43:9-20.

22)Wu MC, Chang YC, Wang TG, Lin LC: Evaluating swallowing dysfunction using a 100-mL water swallowing test. Dysphagia 2004; 19:43-47.

23)Oguchi K, Saitoh E, Baba M, Kusuda S, Tanaka T, Ono K: The repetitive saliva swallowing test (RSST) as a screening test of functional dysphagia (2) Validity of RSST. The Japanese Journal of Rehabilitation Medicine 2000; 37:375-382.

24)Miura H, Hara S, Morisaki N, Yamasaki K. Relationship between comprehensive quality of life and factors related to chewing and swallowing function among community-dwelling elderly individuals. Japanese Journal of Geriatrics 2013 ;

50 : 110-115.

25)Kikutani T, Tamura F, Nishiwaki K, Kodama M, Suda M, Fukui T, et al.: Oral
motor function and masticatory performance in the community-dwelling elderly.
Odontology 2009; 97:38-42.

26)Tsuga K, Yoshida M, Urabe H, Hayashi R, Yoshikawa M, Utanohara Y, et al.:
Effect of general condition and tongue pressure on meal form selection for
elderly care recipient. Journal of Japanese Society for Masticatory Science and
Health Promotion 2004 ; 14:62-67.

27)Kikutani T, Tamura F, Suda M, Kayanaka H, Nishiwaki K, Ino Y, et al.: Effects
of functional oral health care for lingual functions in elderly people requiring
long-term care. Japan Journal of Gerodontology 2005; 19:300-306.

28)Okuno N, Yamamoko K, Akamatu N, Morito M: A study on evaluation of the oral
function in elderly persons. Tsurumi University Dental Journal 2013; 39:11-23.

29)Miura H, Kariyasu M, Sumi Y, Yamasaki K: Labial closure force, activities of
daily living, and cognitive function in frail elderly persons. Japanese Journal of
Geriatrics 2008; 45:520-525.

30)Okada K, Kasiwazaki H, Furuna T, Matusita T, Yamada H, Kanehira T, et al.: The
relationship between nutritional status and oral health status in independent
elderly people—Part 1: A survey before intervention program for sarcopenia.
Japan Journal of Gerodontology 2012; 27:61-68.

31)Tomita K, Okano T, Tamura F, Mukai Y: The relationship between labial
pressure during swallowing and maximum labial pressure-A comparison of
adults and elderly subjects. The Japanese Journal of Dysphagia Rehabilitation
2002; 6:19-26.

32)Yamaguchi M, Adachi T, Ooishi M, Nakatsuka K, Yokoi I, Yoshinari N, et al.:
Multidirectional lip-closing force in healthy elderly persons: Characteristics of
lip-closing force and its relations with physiques, handgrip strength and dentate
status. Journal of the Japanese Society of Stomatognathic Function 2011;
17:125-134.

33)Nakata T, Urakaw S, Takomoto K, Hori E, Ishikawa A, Konishi H, et al.: Effects
of lip closure training on lip functions and brain hemodynamic responses in
healthy female subjects. The Japanese Journal of Dysphagia Rehabilitation
2013; 17:117-125.

34)Nakata T, Urakaw S, Takomoto K, Hori E, Konishi H, Ono T, et al.: Effects of lip
closure training on lip and feeding functions, and diurnal rhythm: A preliminary
research at health care facilities for the elderly. The Japanese Journal of

Dysphagia Rehabilitation 2013; 17:126-133.

35)Nakomura S, Takahashi S, Maeda K, Tanaka Y, Tanino N: The effects of intervention relating to care prevention in the elderly living alone in the community—The effects and utility of full-body and other exercises to enhance the occlusal force. Japan Journal of Gerodontology 2012; 27:311-322.

36)Kono R: Relationship between occlusal force and preventive factors for disability among community-dwelling elderly persons. Japanese Journal of Geriatrics 2009; 46:55-62.

37)Miura H, Watanabe S, Ishigai E, Miura K: Comparison of maximum bite force and dentate status between healthy and frail elderly persons. Journal Of Oral Rehabilitation 2001; 28:592-595.

38)Hare S, Miura H, Yamazaki K, Sumi Y: Association between activities of daily living and oral diadochokinesis among Japanese elderly individuals in a nursing home. Japanese Journal of Geriatrics 2012; 49:330-335.

39)Hara S, Miura H, Yamasaki K: Oral diadochokinesis among Japanese aged over 55 years: analysis of standard values. Japan Journal of Gerodontology 2013; 50:258 -263.

40)Morisaki N, Hiroko M, Usui Y, Moriya S, Hara S: Relationship between oral function and the ability to touch the tip of the tongue to the corners of the mouth among community-dwelling dependent elderly individuals. Japan Journal of Gerodontology 2014; 29:36-41.

41)Parvinen T, Parvinen L, Larmas M: Stimulated salivary flow rate, pH and lactobacillus and yeast concentrations in medicated persons. Scandinavian Journal of Dental Research 1984; 92:524-532.

42)Percival RS, Challacombe SJ, Marsh PD: Flow rates of resting whole and stimulated parotid saliva in relation to age and gender. Journal of Dental Research 1994; 73:1416-1420.

43)Matsuno T, Nakagawa Y, Toya S, Yamaguchi A, Kitahara K, Sato T, et al.: Clinical study on the relationship between dry mouth and long-term medication in elderly patients and its management. Journal of the Japanese Association for Dental Science 2012; 31:49-53.

44)Okamoto M, Kamoi M, Tsurumoto A, Yamachika S, Imamura T, Yamamoto K, et al.: Quantitative evaluation of candida by microscopy. Japanese Journal of Oral and Maxillofacial Surgery 2012; 61:33-38.

45)Morisaki N, Miura H: Detection and analysis of influential factors related to opportunistically infecting microorganisms in the oral cavity among disabled elderly individuals in geriatric health service. Facilities Japan Journal of Gerodontology 2010; 25:289-296.

46)Sato T, Tanaka T, Yaegaki K: Comparison of the oral flora of independent elderly and those requiring nursing assistance . Dentistry in Japan 2006; 42:86-89.

47)Hirota K, Yoneyama T, Ota M, et al.: Pharyngeal bacteria and professional oral health care in elderly people. Japanese Journal of Geriatrics 1997; 34:125-129.

48)Adachi M, Ishihara K, Abe S, Okuda K, Ishikawa T: Effect of professional oral health care on elderly living in nursing homes. Oral Sur Oral Med Oral Pathol Oral Radiol Endod 2002; 94:191-195.

49)Morisaki N, Miura H, Moriya S, Hara S: Relationship between the swallowing function and the health-related QOL among community-dwelling dependent elderly persons. Japanese Journal of Geriatrics 2014; 51:259-263.

50)Tomita K, Ishikawa K, Niiya H, Sekiguchi H, Mukai Y: The transition of the effect of oral function training program in the Elderly. Japanese Journal of Gerodontology 2007; 5:31-35.

51)Sakashita R, Watanabe K, Nishihira T, Arai K, Matsushita K, Yamakawa T, et al.: Community health promotion program focusing on oral health for elderly people at a district. University of Hyogo College of Nursing Art and Science Research Institute of Nursing Care for People and Community Bulletin 2011;18:11-22.

52)Serra-Prat M, Palomera M, Gomez C, Sar-Shalom D, Saiz A, Montoya JG: Oropharyngeal dysphagia as a risk factor for malnutrition and lower respiratory tract infection in independently living older persons: a population-based prospective study. Age Ageing 2012; 41:371-381.

53)Takai I, Murakami M, Oonisi M, Nakayama M, Tanaka M, Ochi K, et al.: Risk factors associated with dysphagia among frail elderly. Journal of Physiological Anthropology 2006; 11:127-132.

54)Cabre M, Serra-Prat M, Palomera E, Almirall J, Pallares R, Clave P: Prevalence and prognostic implications of dysphagia in elderly patients with pneumonia. Age Ageing 2010; 39:39-45.

55)Hirayama Y, Otsu C, Komatsu Y, Yoshini M, Ishi Y, Mazaki T, et al.: The usefulness of the Mini-Nutritional Assessment-Short Form for evaluating the nutrition of senior inpatients. Journal of Nihon University Medical Association 2011; 70:203-207.

56)Maruyama T, Kigawa M, Miura A, Shimizu S: A trial of nutritional evaluation by mini nutritional assessment (MNA) at a welfare facility for the elderly. Japan Society of Nutrition and Food Science 2006; 59:207-213.

57)Sugiyama T, Ohkubo M, Honda Y, Tasaki A, Nagasawa K, Ishida R, et al: Effect of swallowing exercises in independent elderly. The Bulletin of Tokyo Dental College 2013; 54:109-115.

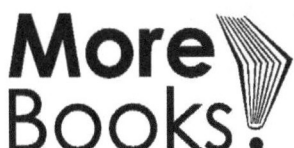
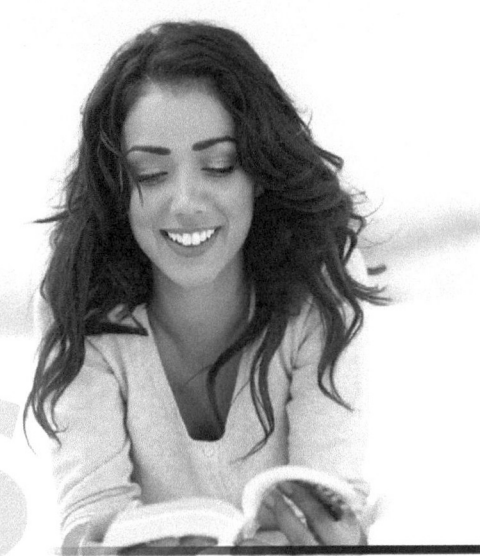
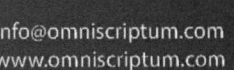 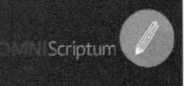

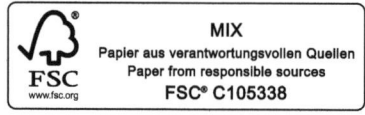